To: Araela & Price,
Love, aunt Maxine

7-2023

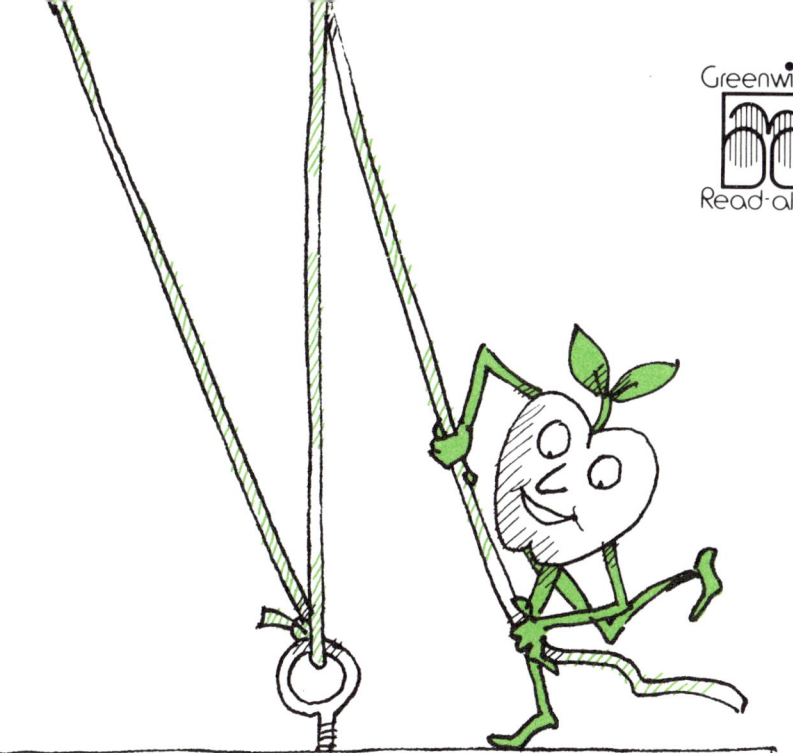

Greenwillow Read-alone

VITAMINS
What They Are, What They Do

by JUDITH S. SEIXAS
illustrated by TOM HUFFMAN

GREENWILLOW BOOKS · NEW YORK

Text copyright © 1986
by Judith S. Seixas
Illustrations copyright © 1986
by Tom Huffman
All rights reserved.
No part of this book may be
reproduced or utilized in any
form or by any means, electronic
or mechanical, including
photocopying, recording or by
any information storage and
retrieval system, without
permission in writing from the
Publisher, Greenwillow Books,
a division of
William Morrow & Company, Inc.,
1350 Avenue of the Americas,
New York, NY 10019.
Printed in the
United States of America
First Edition
10 9 8 7 6 5 4 3 2

Library of Congress
Cataloging-in-Publication Data
Seixas, Judith S.
Vitamins: what they are, what they do.
Summary: Discusses vitamins,
how they were discovered,
how they work, how they can be made,
and how they fit into our diets.
1. Vitamins—Juvenile literature.
[1. Vitamins]
I. Huffman, Tom, ill.   II. Title.
QP771.S45   1986   613.2'8
85-17761   ISBN 0-688-06065-X
ISBN 0-688-06066-8 (lib. bdg.)

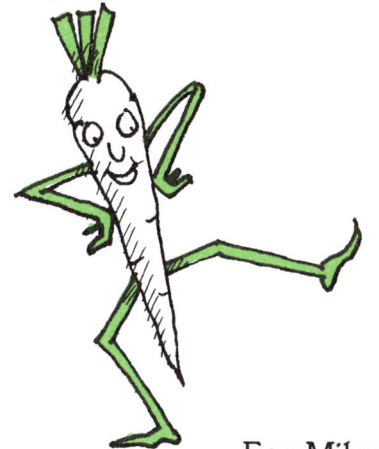

For Mikaela Judith—
with love
from her grandma
—J. S. S.

For Little Momma May
—T. H.

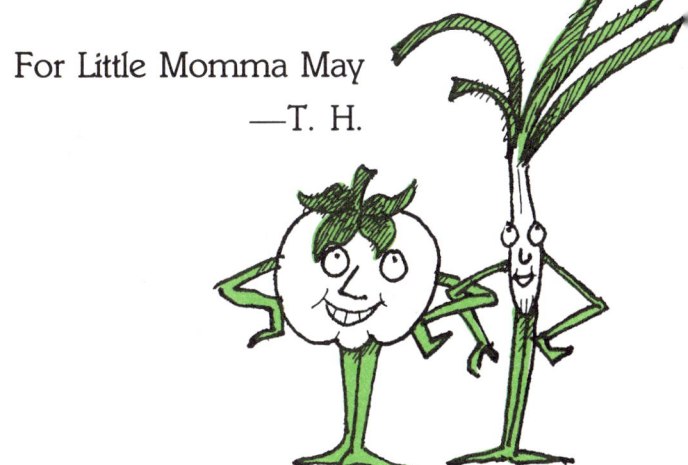

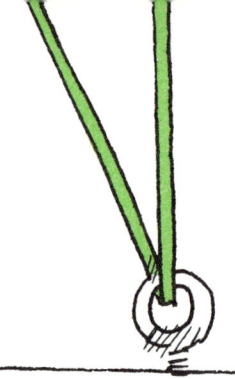

Contents

Introduction 6
1. What Are Vitamins? 8
2. How Vitamins Were Discovered 10
3. "A, B, C . . ." 19
4. How Vitamins Work 24
5. How Vitamins Are Made 31

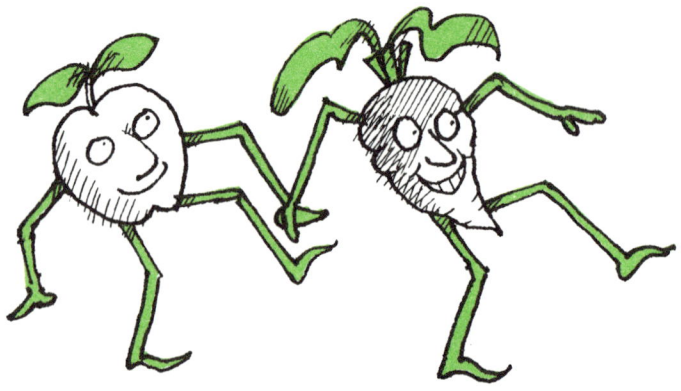

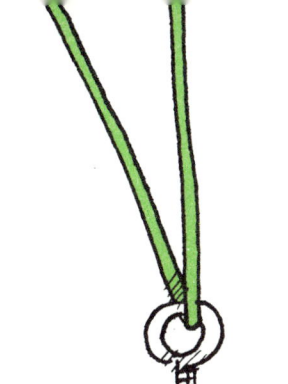

6. Enriched Food 36
7. Reading Labels 39
8. A Balanced Diet 41
   Conclusion 48
   VITAMIN CHART 52
   VITAMIN TEST 54

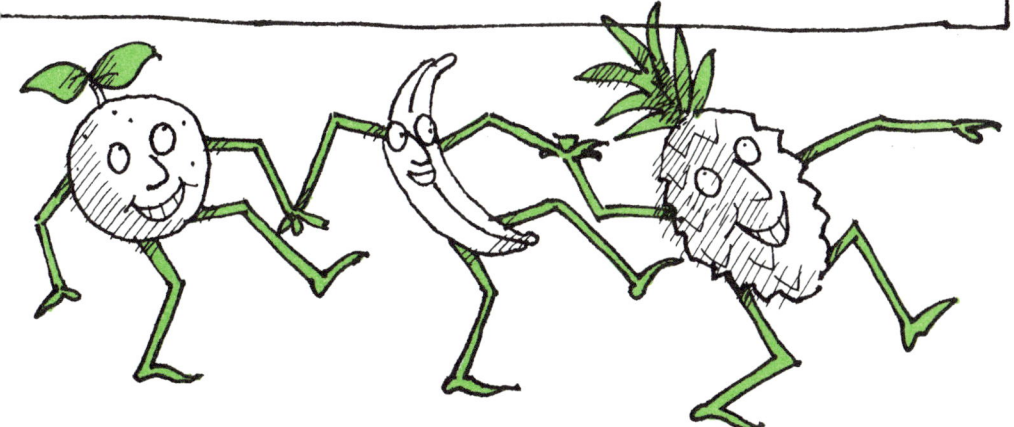

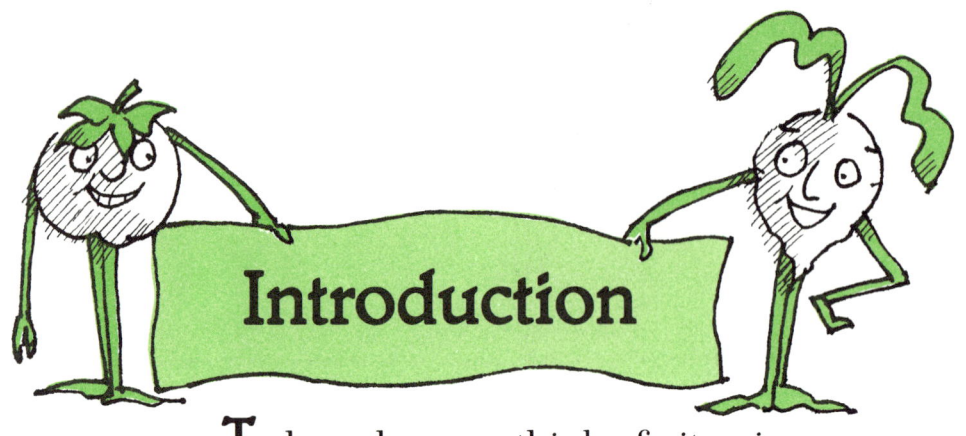

Introduction

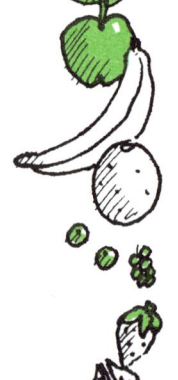

Today when we think of vitamins, we think of pills and capsules. But these man-made vitamins were not known before the 1930s. For thousands of years people got all the vitamins they needed from the foods they ate. They ate mostly fresh fruits, berries, nuts, vegetables, and meat. They did not eat junk food, which has little food value.

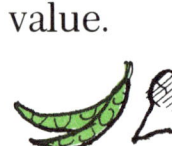

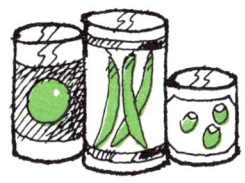

They did not eat canned
or frozen foods.
We know that when food
is canned, cooked, or frozen,
many vitamins are lost.
Because of the way we eat today,
many people add vitamins
to their diet.
They take vitamin pills
or capsules.
They choose enriched
or fortified foods to which
vitamins have been added.

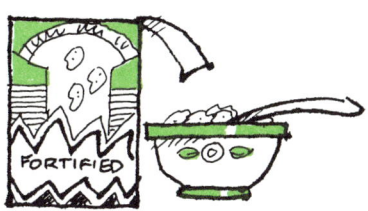

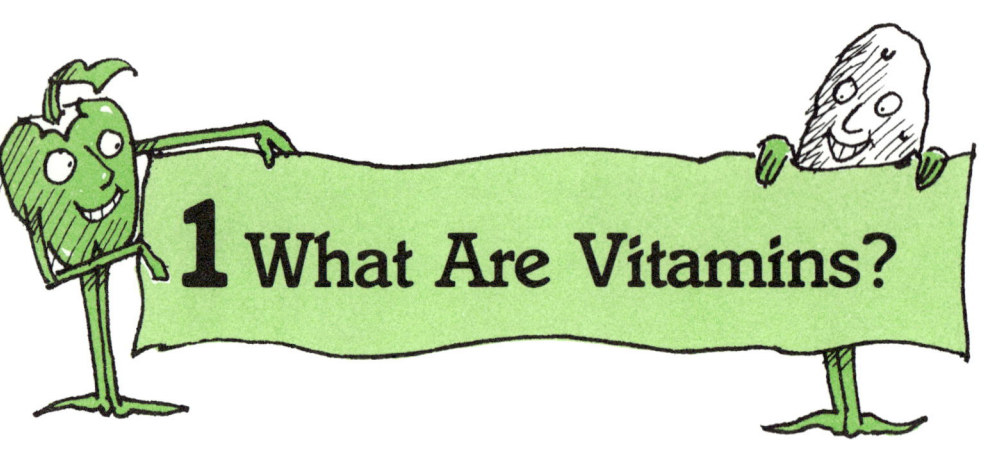

1 What Are Vitamins?

Vitamins are chemicals
found in foods.
You cannot see them.
They are not
in the air you breathe.
They are not
in the water you drink.
Most of them have no taste.

Today there are thirteen
known vitamins.
You need them to grow.
You need them to stay healthy.
You need them to look
and feel your best.
You need them all.
But you need them
only in small amounts.

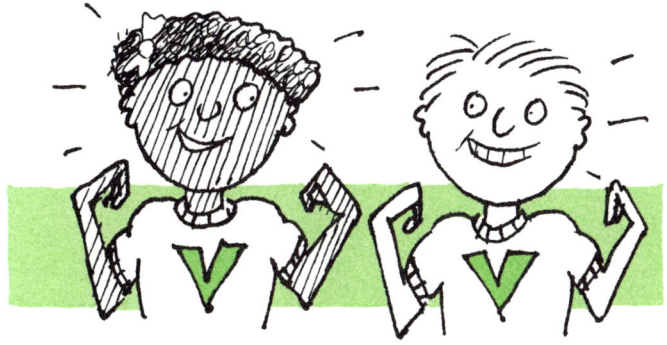

2 How Vitamins Were Discovered

The Search

Years ago sailors who went on long sea voyages developed a strange sickness. Their gums bled, their teeth fell out, their skin bruised easily. They became weak. Some even died. The sickness was called SCURVY. In about 1740, Dr. James Lind, a Scottish ship's doctor, made a discovery.

He found that sailors
who stopped at tropical islands
where they could eat citrus fruits
were cured of their scurvy.
Citrus fruits also prevented others
from getting scurvy.

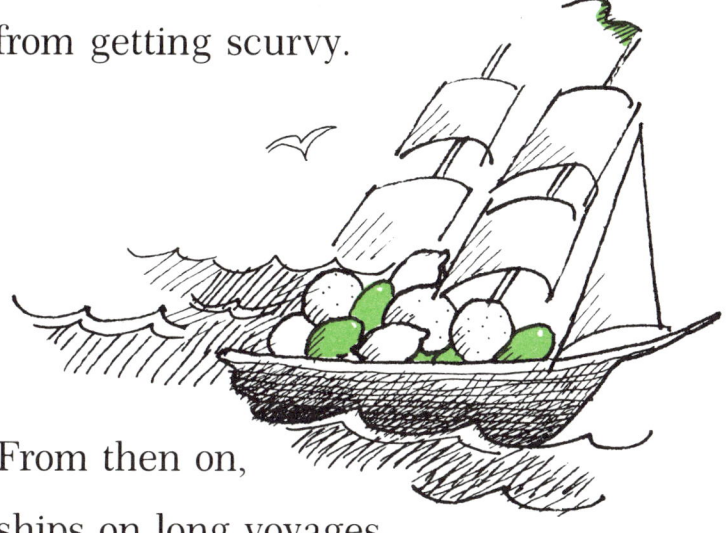

From then on,
ships on long voyages
made sure to carry a good supply
of lemons, oranges, and limes.
That is why British sailors
came to be known as limeys.

The cure for scurvy
had been found, but
the *cause* was still a mystery.
Scientists searched for it
in polluted water.
They looked for it in rotted foods.
They looked for a scurvy germ.
They looked for poisons.
It became clear
that scurvy was not caused
by something the sailors ate.
The search had come
to a dead end.

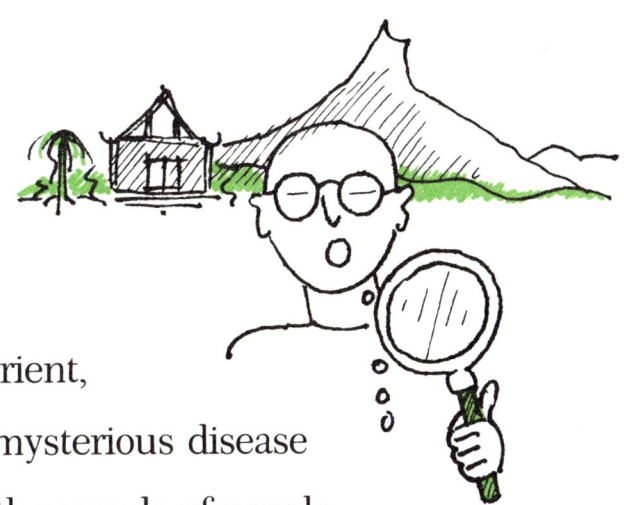

In the Orient,
another mysterious disease
affected thousands of people.
It was called BERIBERI.
Like scurvy, its cause was unknown.
It was not until 1882
that a Japanese scientist
found the clue.
The basic food of Oriental people
was white rice.
He found that meat and vegetables
added to white rice diets
prevented beriberi.

13

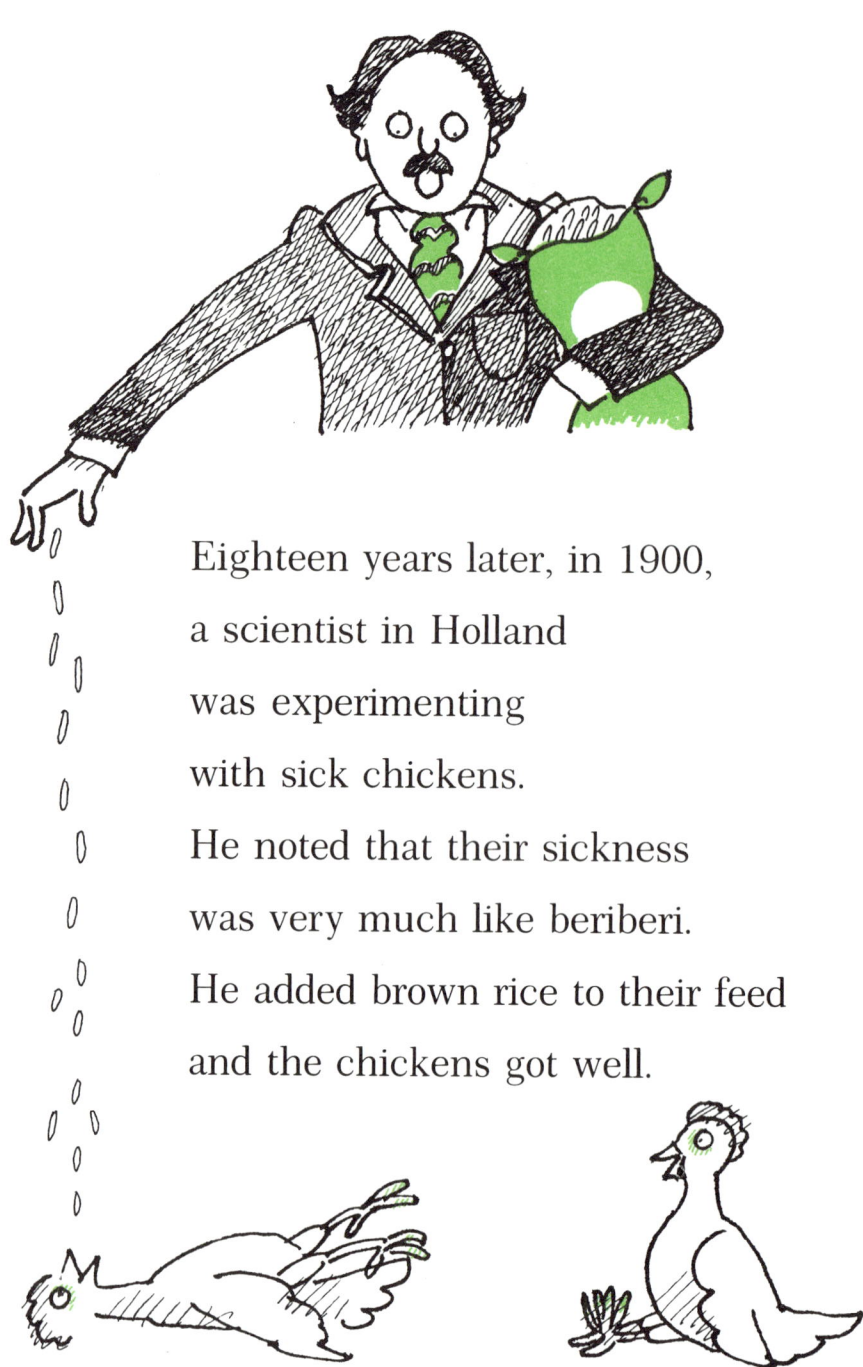

Eighteen years later, in 1900,
a scientist in Holland
was experimenting
with sick chickens.
He noted that their sickness
was very much like beriberi.
He added brown rice to their feed
and the chickens got well.

He then found that
people who ate whole rice,
which included the brown husks,
did not get beriberi.
He became convinced
that a substance in rice husks
could prevent beriberi.
But, like Dr. Lind, he did not know
what caused the illness.
By now scientists the world over
were looking for an answer.

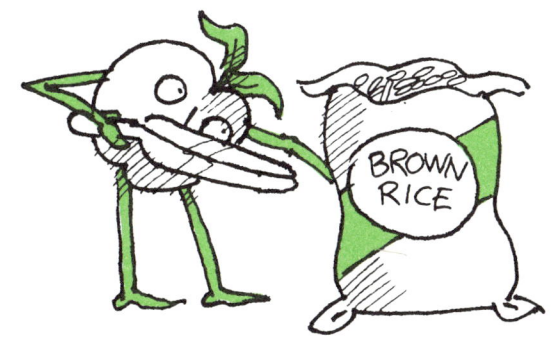

15

In 1912 a Polish doctor
tried to separate
the "anti-beriberi factor"
from rice husks.
And in England a fellow scientist
was working on the same problem.
Finally both scientists
came to the same conclusion.

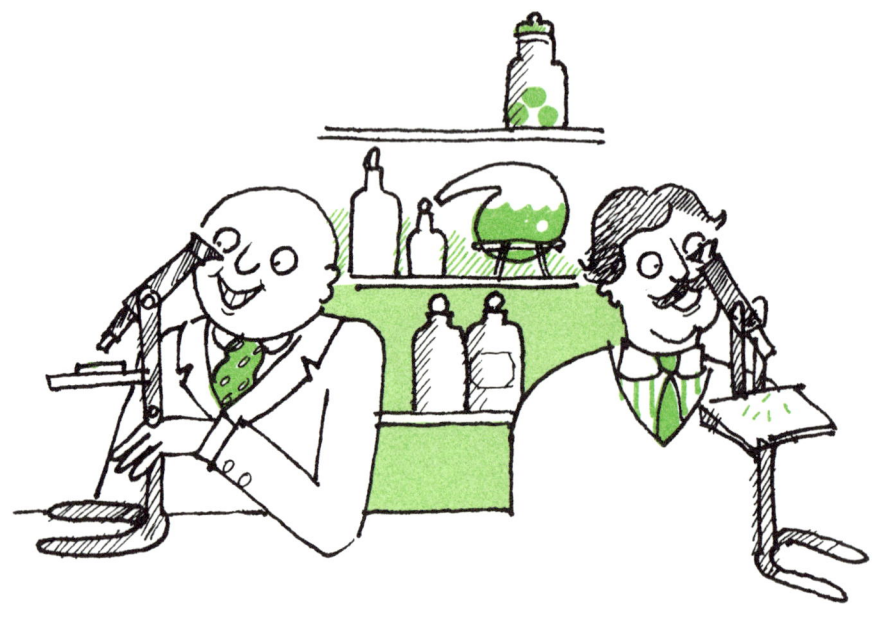

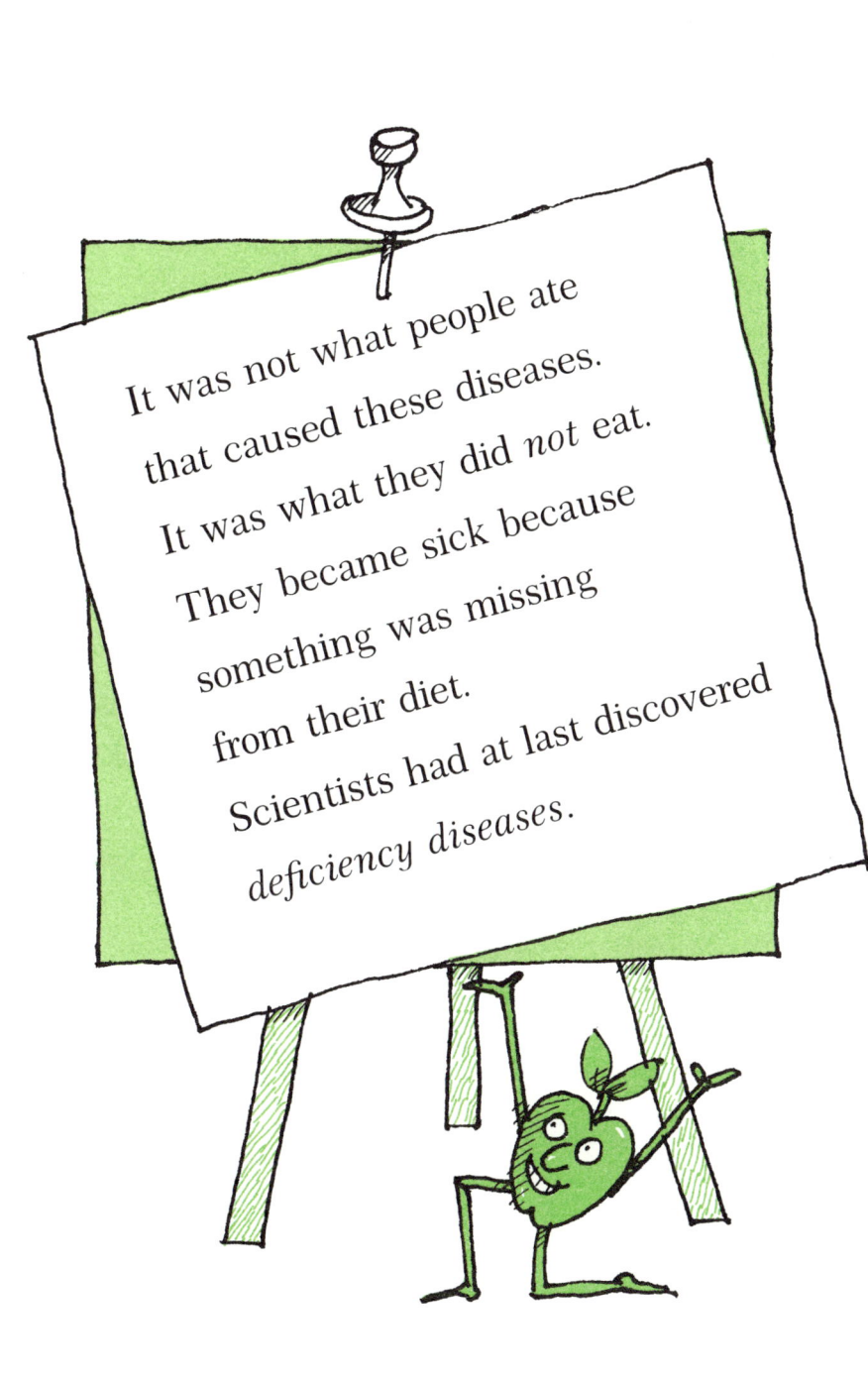

Deficiency Diseases

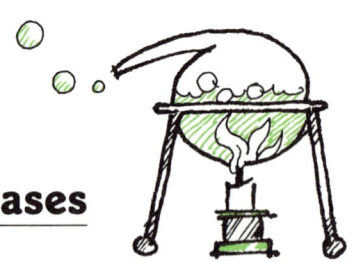

Soon two other deficiency diseases were found.

One was RICKETS.

Its main symptom is softening of the bones.

The other was PELLAGRA.

Its main symptoms are itching, red skin, and general weakness.

A corrected diet could prevent or cure these illnesses.

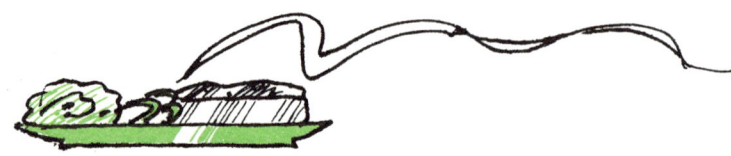

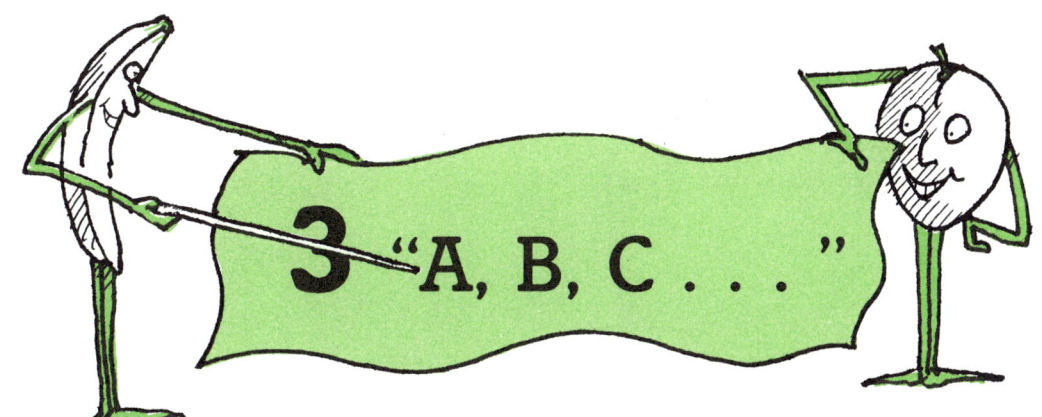

3 "A, B, C..."

The First Vitamins

In 1913 scientists discovered chemical substances they called vitamins. The first ones were named Vitamin A and Vitamin B.

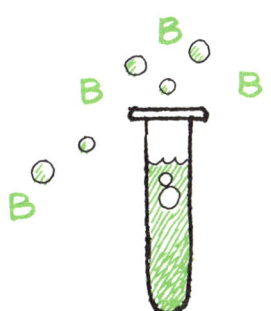

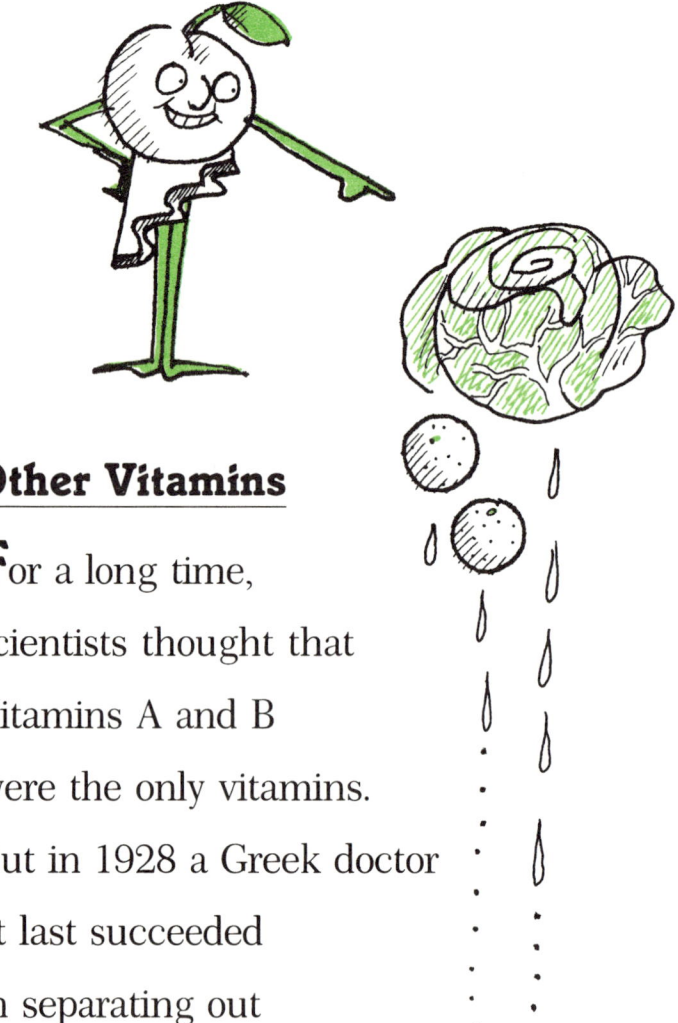

Other Vitamins

For a long time,
scientists thought that
Vitamins A and B
were the only vitamins.
But in 1928 a Greek doctor
at last succeeded
in separating out
a white powder from oranges
and cabbages.

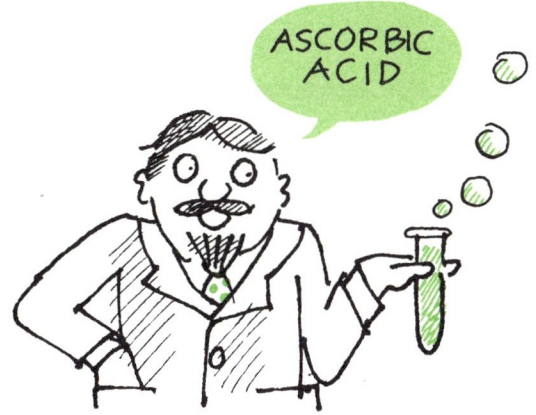

This white powder was
the substance that cured scurvy.
He called it ascorbic acid.
Ascorbic comes from
a Greek word
meaning "no scurvy."
Now ascorbic acid is also
known as Vitamin C.
Other vitamins were soon discovered.
Vitamin B_{12} was found in 1948.
No new vitamin has been found
since then.

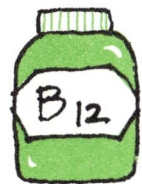

The thirteen known vitamins are divided into two classes: water-soluble and fat-soluble.

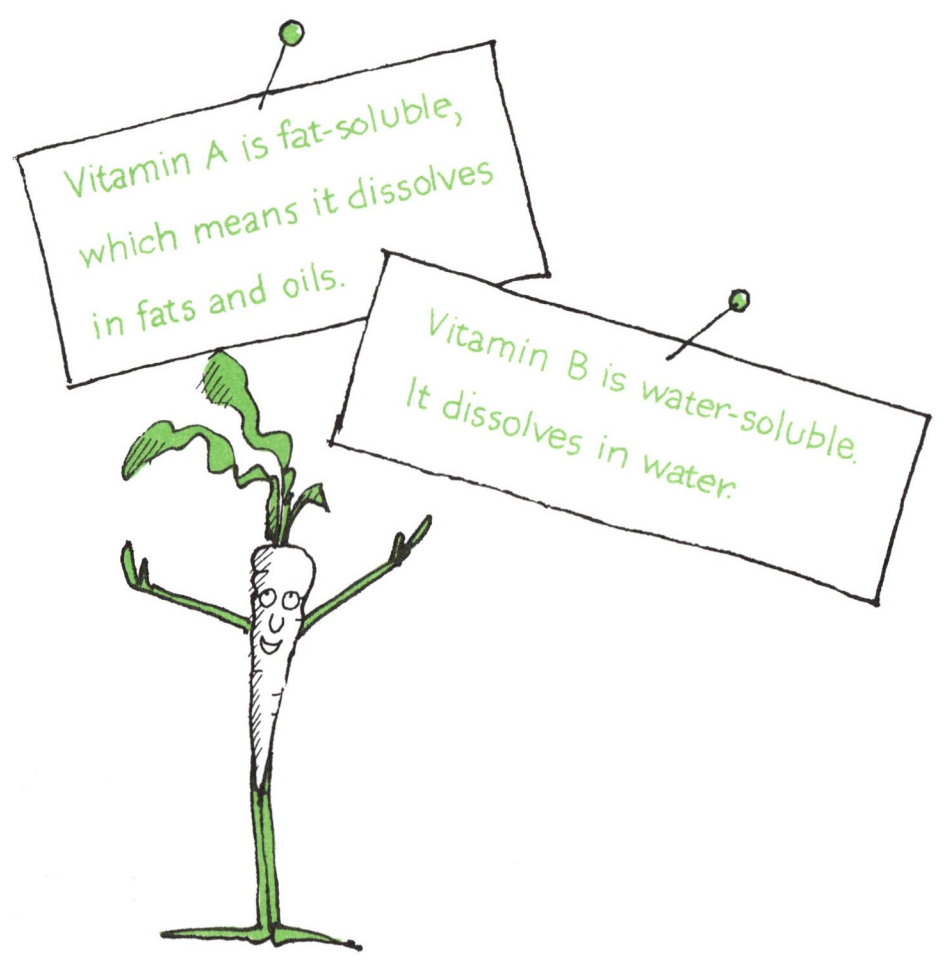

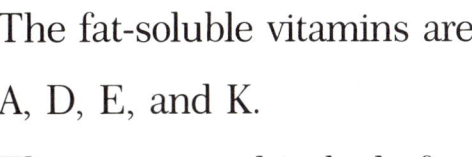

The fat-soluble vitamins are
A, D, E, and K.
They are stored in body fat.

The water-soluble vitamins are
the Vitamin B family:
B_1 (thiamine); B_2 (riboflavin);
B_3 (niacin); B_6 (pyridoxine);
B_{12} (cobalomine);
biotin;
pantothenic acid;
folic acid;
and Vitamin C.

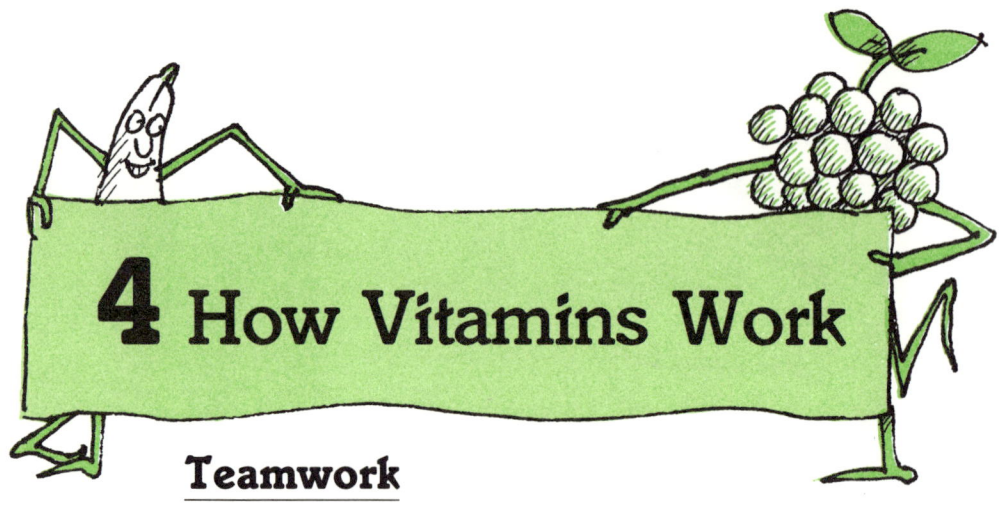

4 How Vitamins Work

Teamwork

Vitamins work as a team.

Each one has its tasks.

Each one has its place.

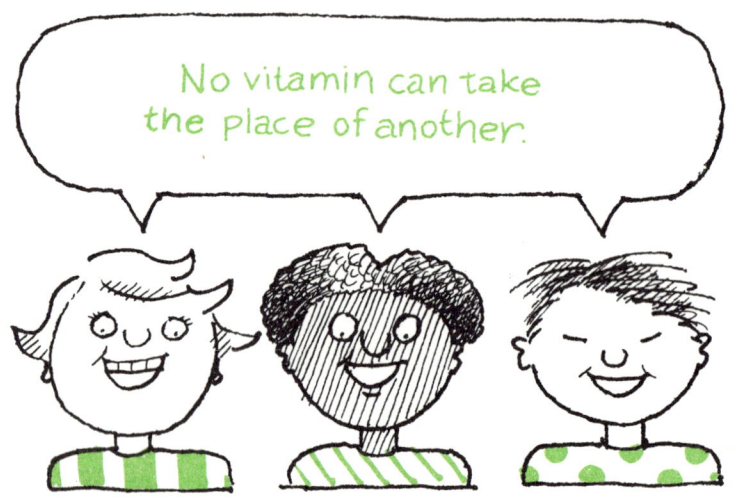

True vitamins keep the
teamwork going.
These are known as *catalysts*.
If one is missing,
the others don't work as well.
At one time, some substances
were thought to be vitamins.
But they did not work with the team.
Therefore, they were not
true vitamins.

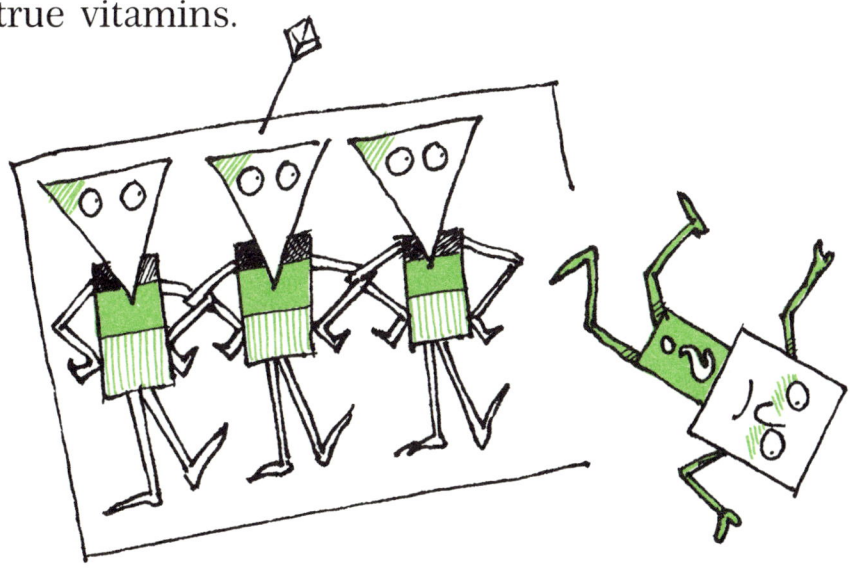

What Each Vitamin Does

VITAMIN A

affects how well
we see in dim light.
It helps keep skin, nails,
and hair healthy.

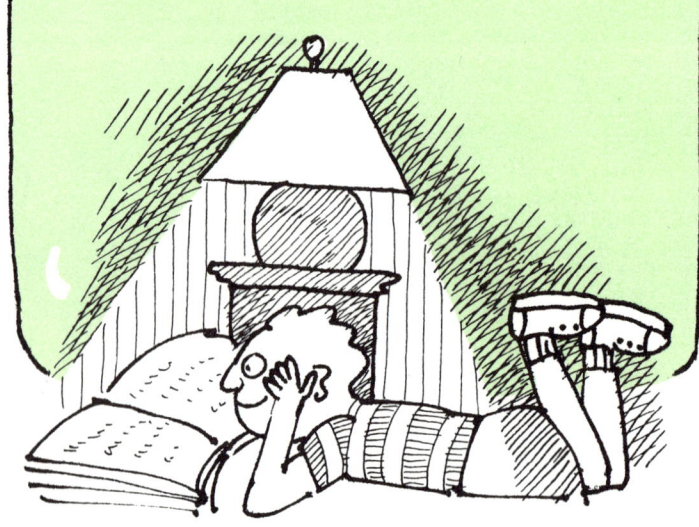

The VITAMIN B FAMILY

builds body cells.
It keeps the nervous system
and digestive tract working well.
It also keeps blood, skin,
and hair healthy.
The B vitamins are known as
the *B family* or *B complex*
because they are found in many
of the same foods.
As we know, Vitamin B
prevents beriberi and pellagra.

VITAMIN C

is needed

to build strong muscles,

body cells, and blood vessels.

It prevents scurvy.

Humans, monkeys, apes,

and guinea pigs

must get their Vitamin C

from what they eat.

Other animals make it

in their own bodies.

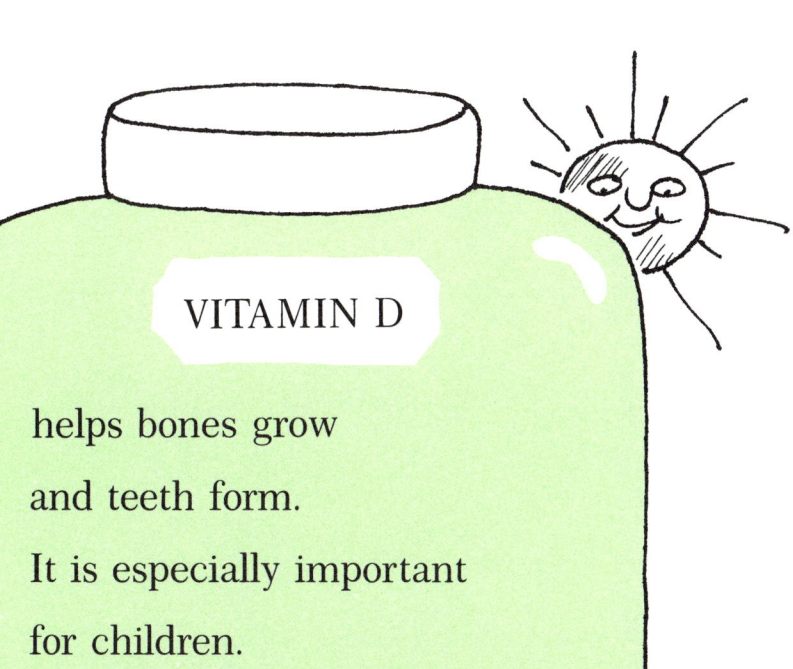

VITAMIN D

helps bones grow
and teeth form.
It is especially important
for children.
It helps the body use calcium
and prevents rickets.
It is known as
the sunshine vitamin
because a substance in our skin
is made into Vitamin D in
daylight.

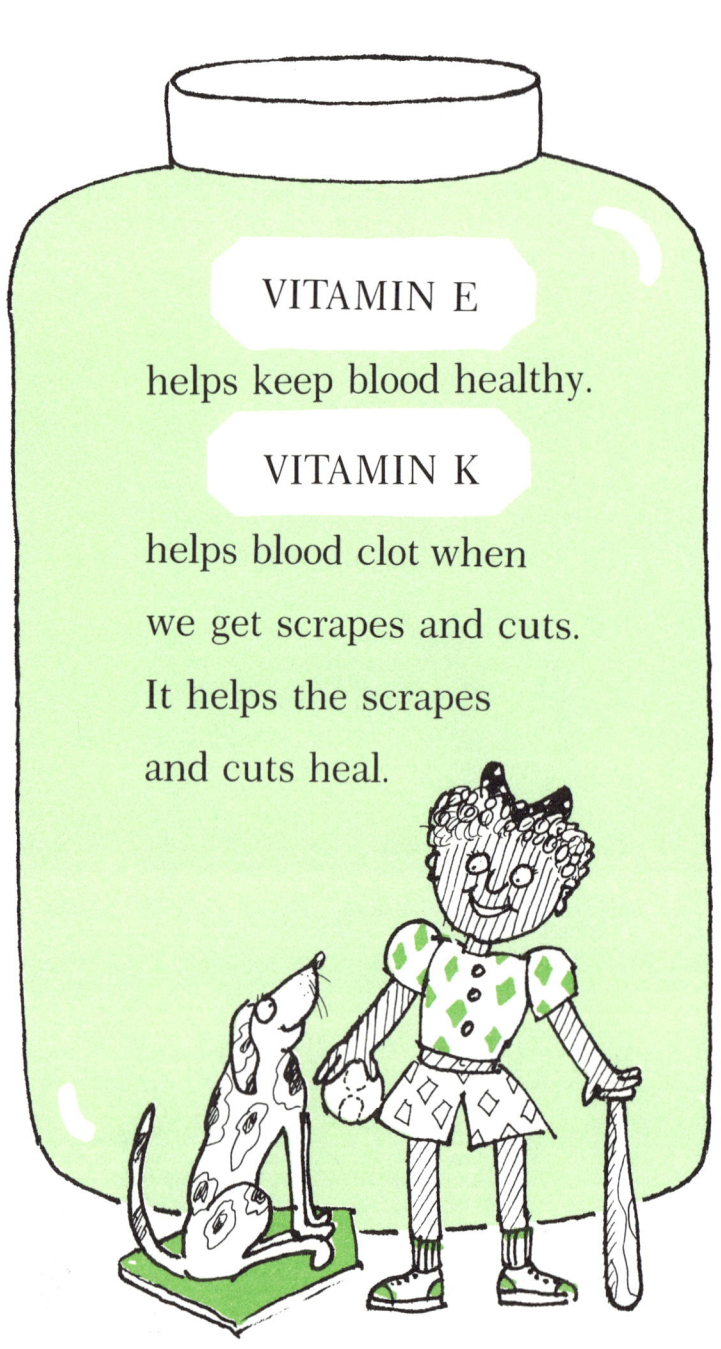

VITAMIN E

helps keep blood healthy.

VITAMIN K

helps blood clot when we get scrapes and cuts. It helps the scrapes and cuts heal.

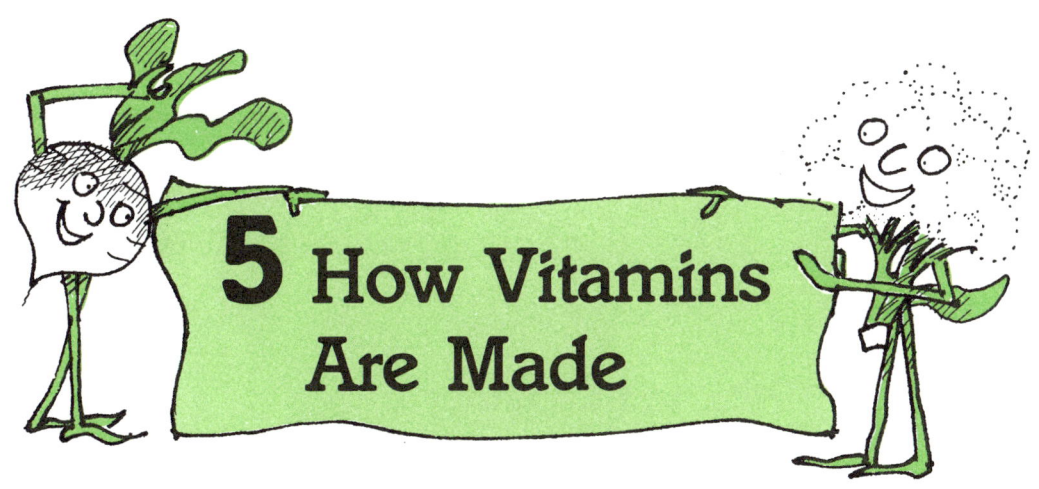

5 How Vitamins Are Made

Man-made Vitamins

In the 1930s chemists learned how to separate pure vitamins from food. We call these natural vitamins. They also learned to make them from chemicals. We call these synthetic vitamins. Whether vitamins are natural or synthetic, they are equally good for you.

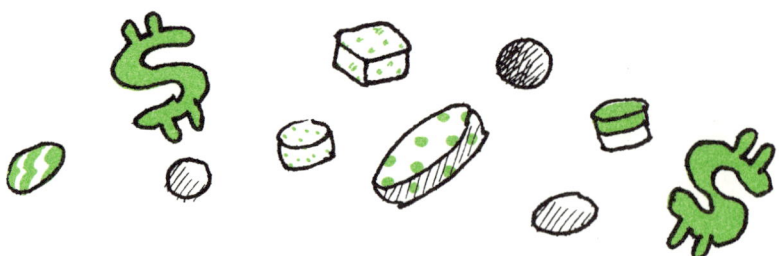

Pills and Capsules

Americans spend two and a half billion dollars buying man-made vitamins each year.
These vitamins come in a rainbow of colors.
They come in fruit flavors.
They come in the shapes of animals
and cartoon characters.
They come in chewables.
They come in liquid drops
and in capsules.

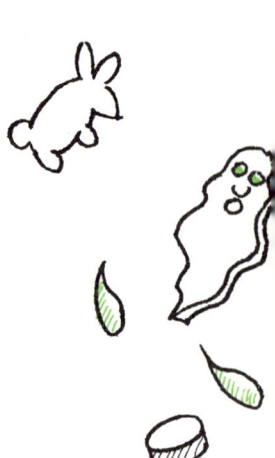

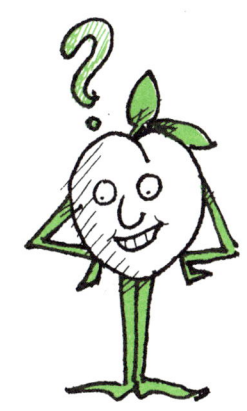

Are Vitamin Pills Safe?

Some people wonder

if vitamin pills are safe.

Others believe

the more you take

the healthier you will be.

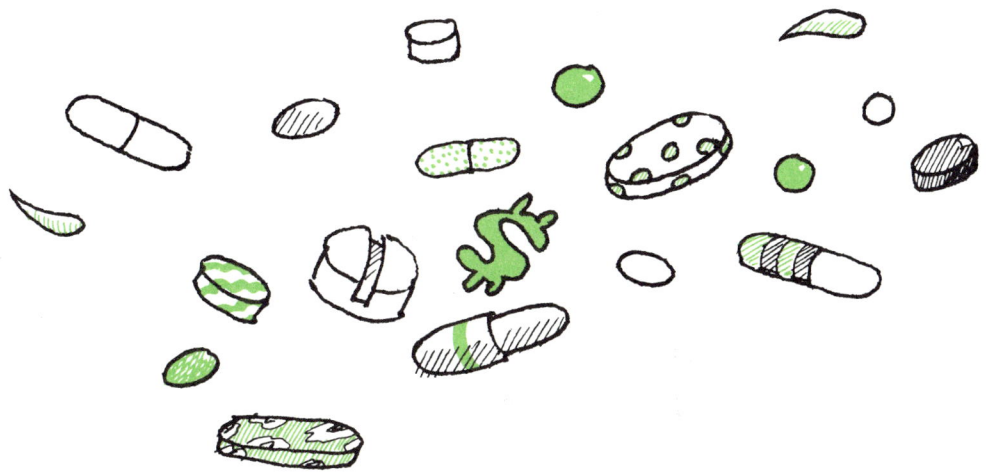

The truth is that too much
of some vitamins can be harmful.
Too much can cause stomach aches,
headaches, dry skin, hair loss,
sore lips, deformed bones,
and nerve problems.
Often children like
the taste of vitamins.
But vitamins are not candy!
Too much of some vitamins
can make you sick.

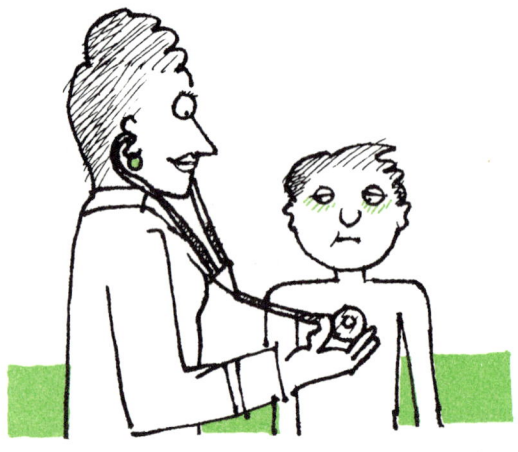

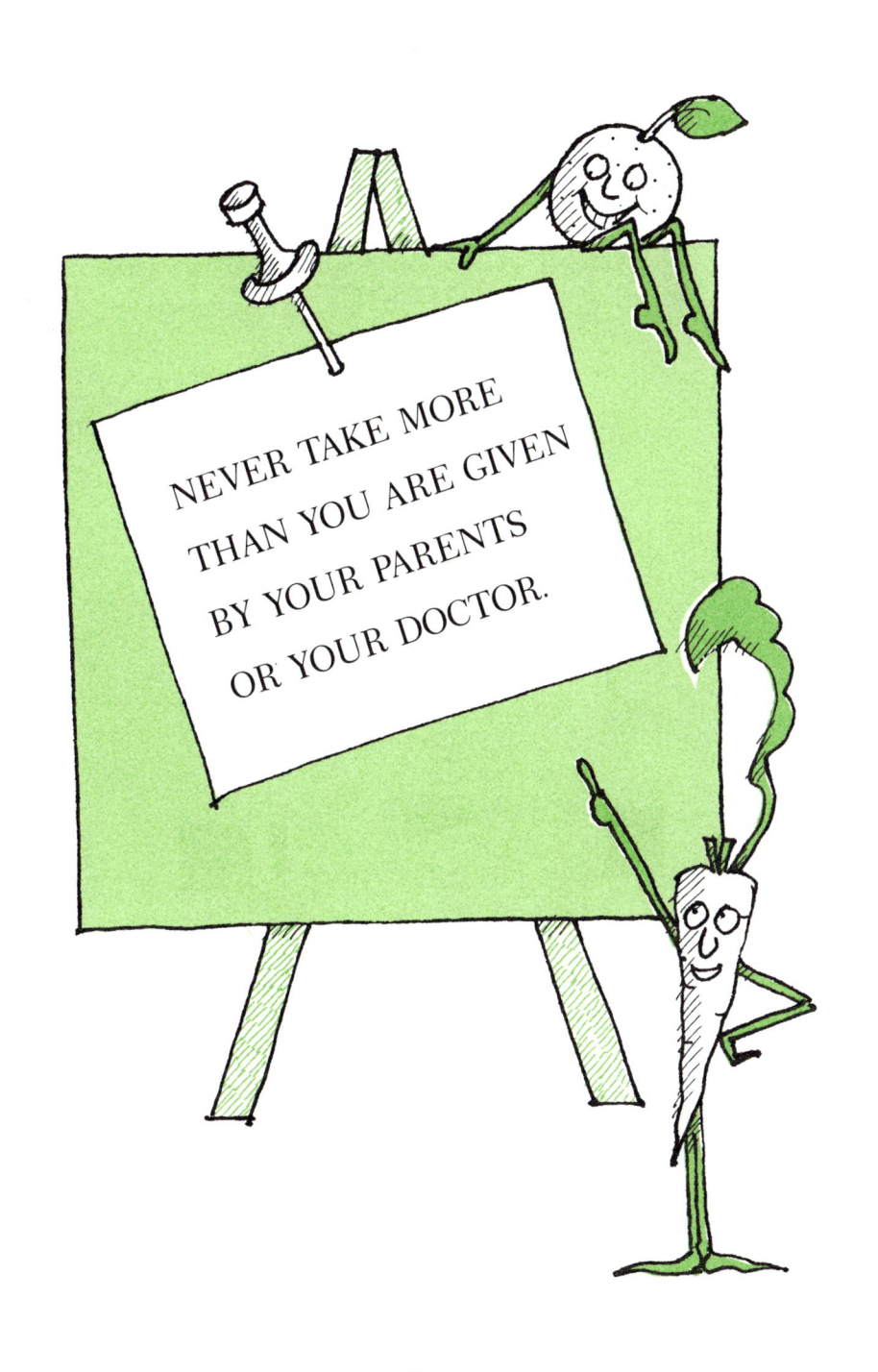

NEVER TAKE MORE THAN YOU ARE GIVEN BY YOUR PARENTS OR YOUR DOCTOR.

6 Enriched Food

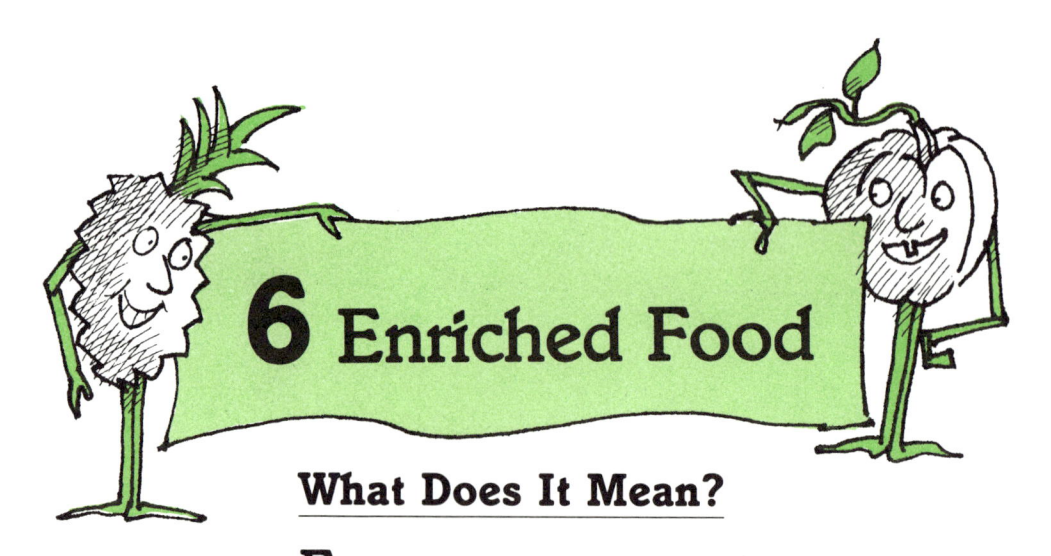

What Does It Mean?

Food can lose vitamins when it is processed. The discovery of how to make vitamins made it possible to add vitamins to processed foods.

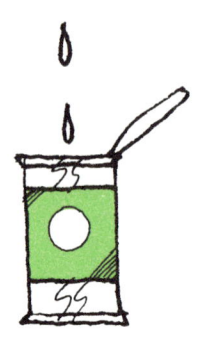

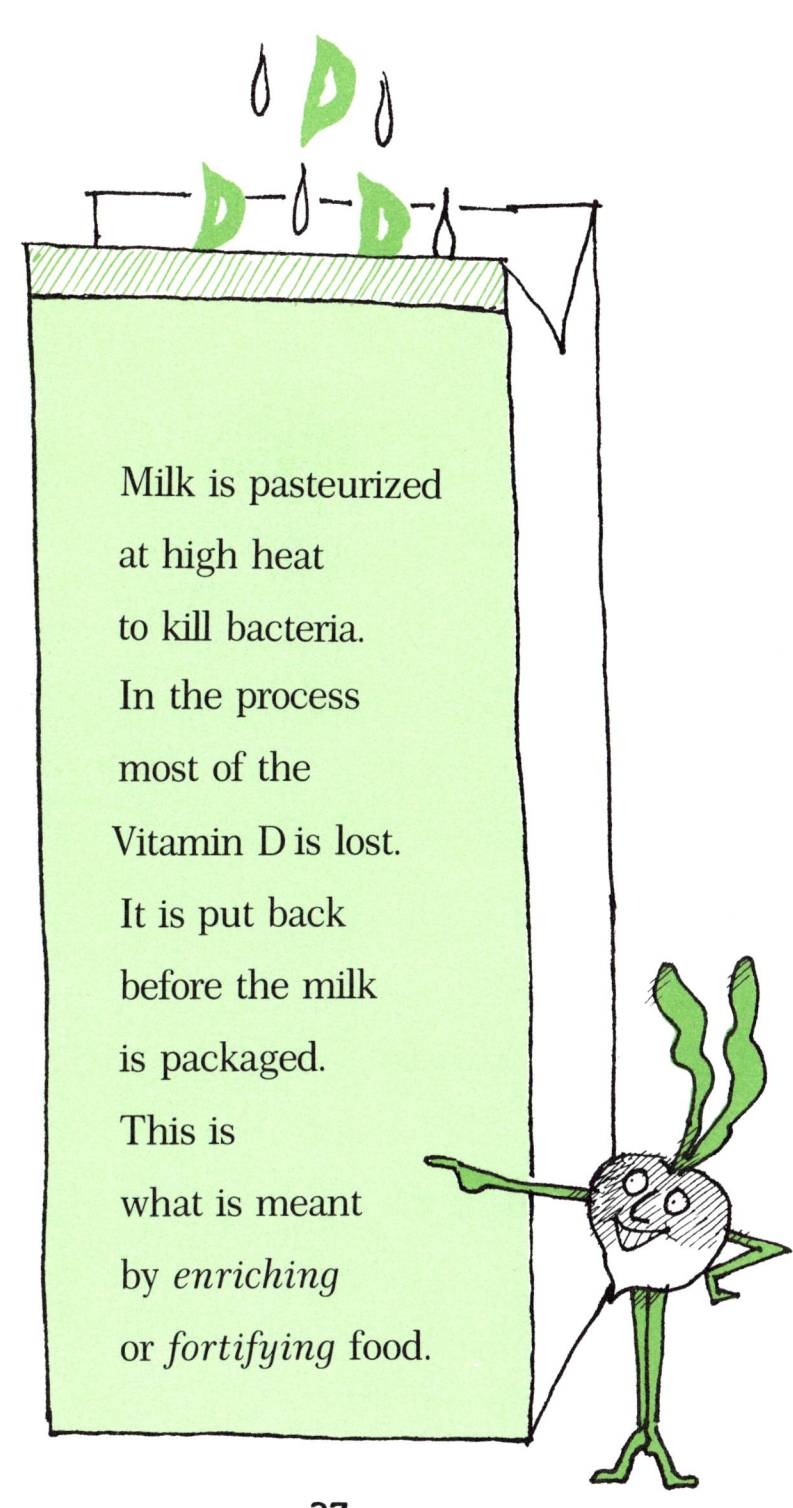

Milk is pasteurized
at high heat
to kill bacteria.
In the process
most of the
Vitamin D is lost.
It is put back
before the milk
is packaged.
This is
what is meant
by *enriching*
or *fortifying* food.

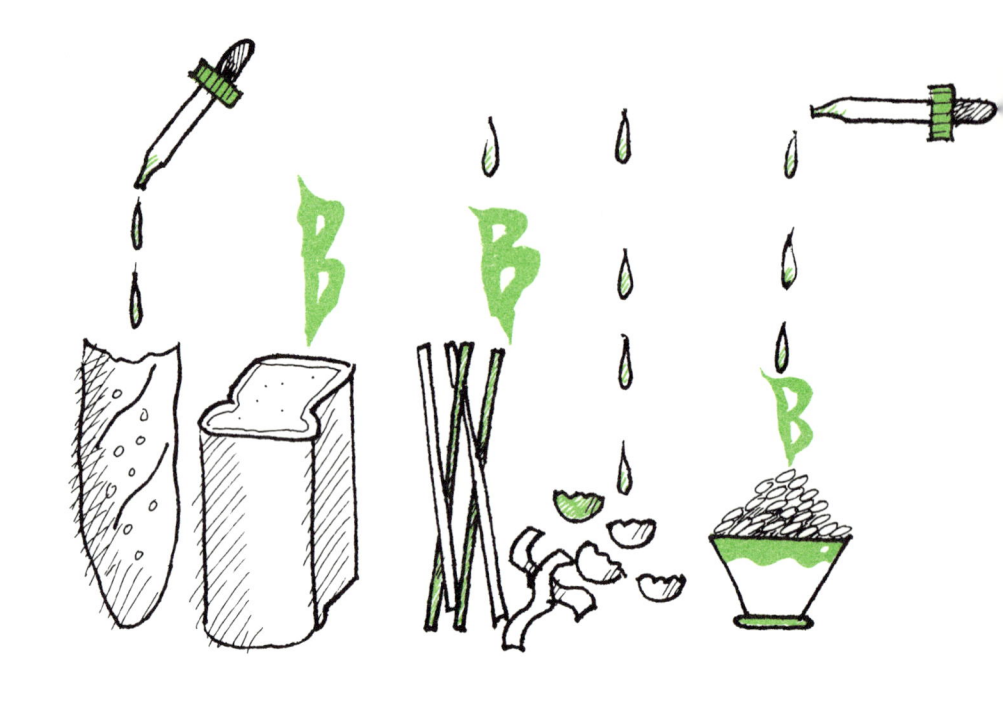

Breads, pastas, and white rice
are enriched
with Vitamin B complex.
Many fruit juices are fortified
with Vitamin C.
Read the labels on food packages.
You will see which vitamins
have been added.

7 Reading Labels

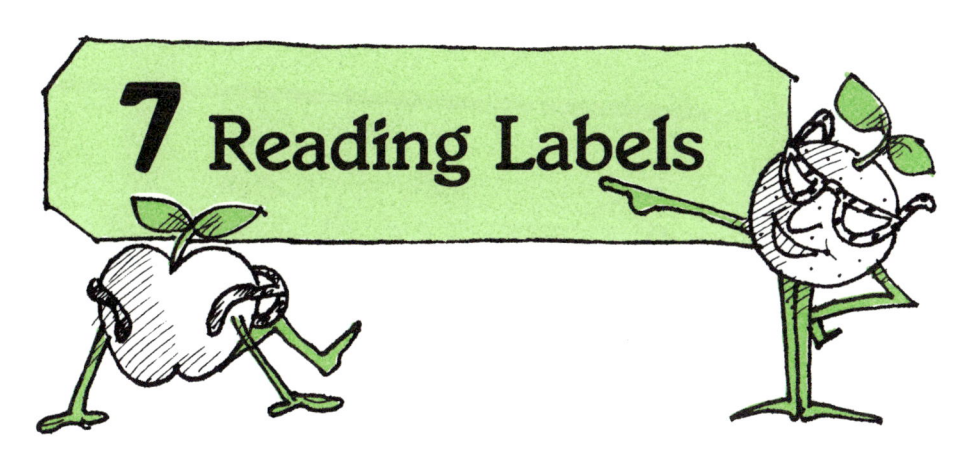

What Do the Lists of Numbers Mean?

What do the lists mean on package labels? They are the daily amounts of vitamins and other nutrients needed by healthy people. These lists must be printed on all packaged foods.

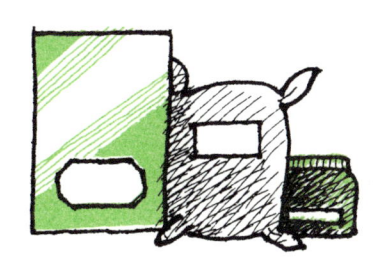

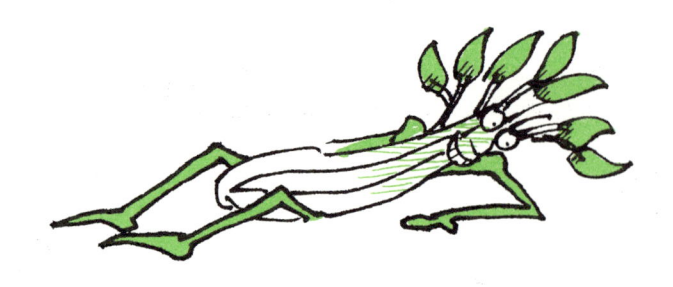

The amounts are based
on findings of the
Food and Nutrition Board of the
National Academy of Sciences.
"The United States Recommended
Dietary Allowances" (RDA)
are shown in this way:

"Vitamin C . . . 10"

This means that one serving
of the food in the package
has one-tenth (10%) of the
Vitamin C you need each day.

8 A Balanced Diet

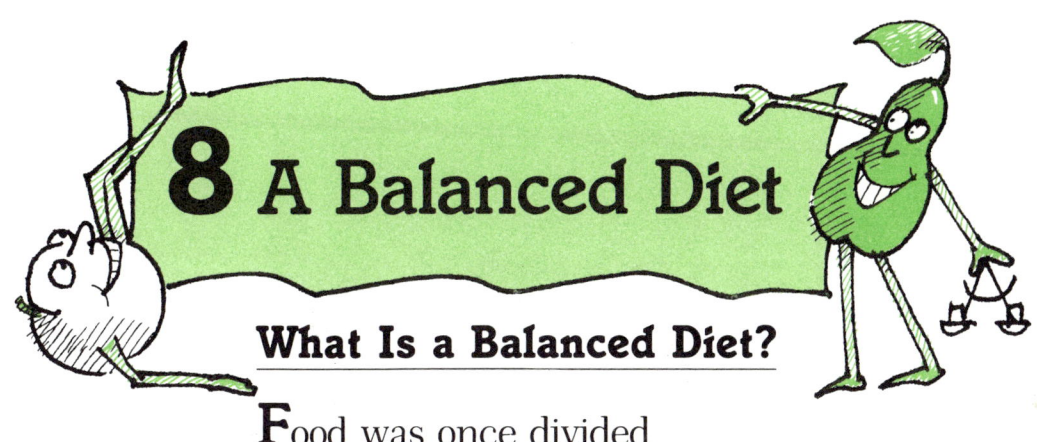

What Is a Balanced Diet?

Food was once divided into four groups.

Now it is divided into six groups:

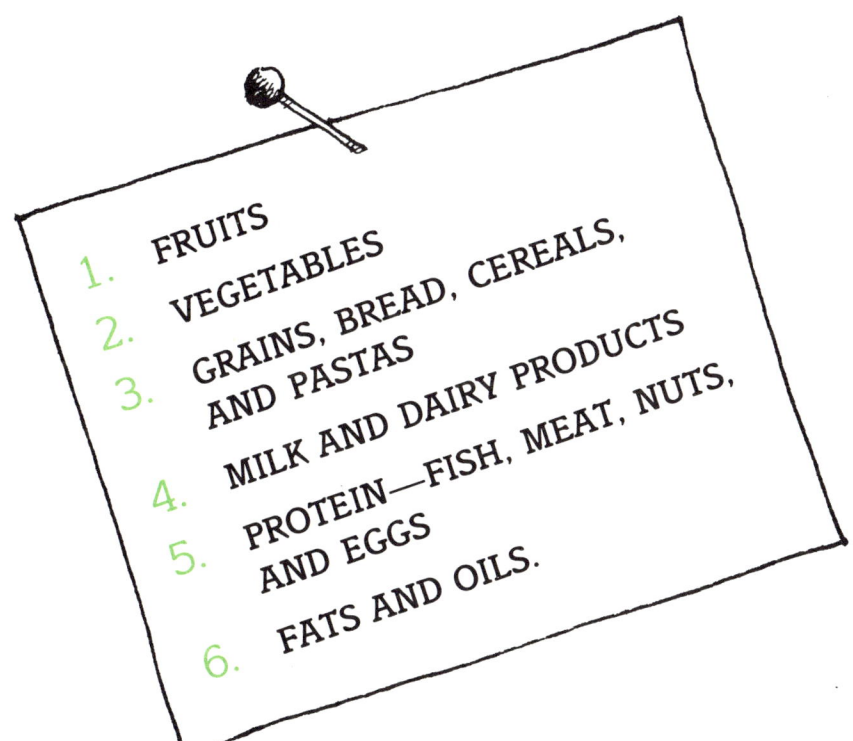

1. FRUITS
2. VEGETABLES
3. GRAINS, BREAD, CEREALS, AND PASTAS
4. MILK AND DAIRY PRODUCTS
5. PROTEIN—FISH, MEAT, NUTS, AND EGGS
6. FATS AND OILS.

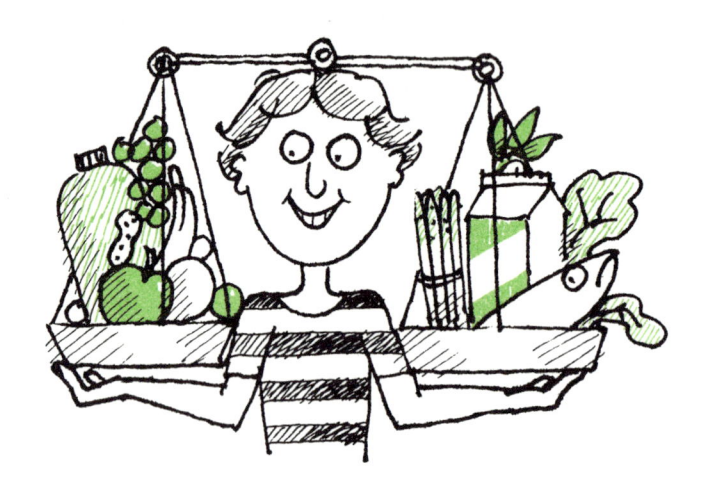

A balanced diet includes food from each of the six groups. You should eat food from each group every day.

The B family and Vitamin C quickly leave the body in urine and perspiration. Therefore, you should have them every day.

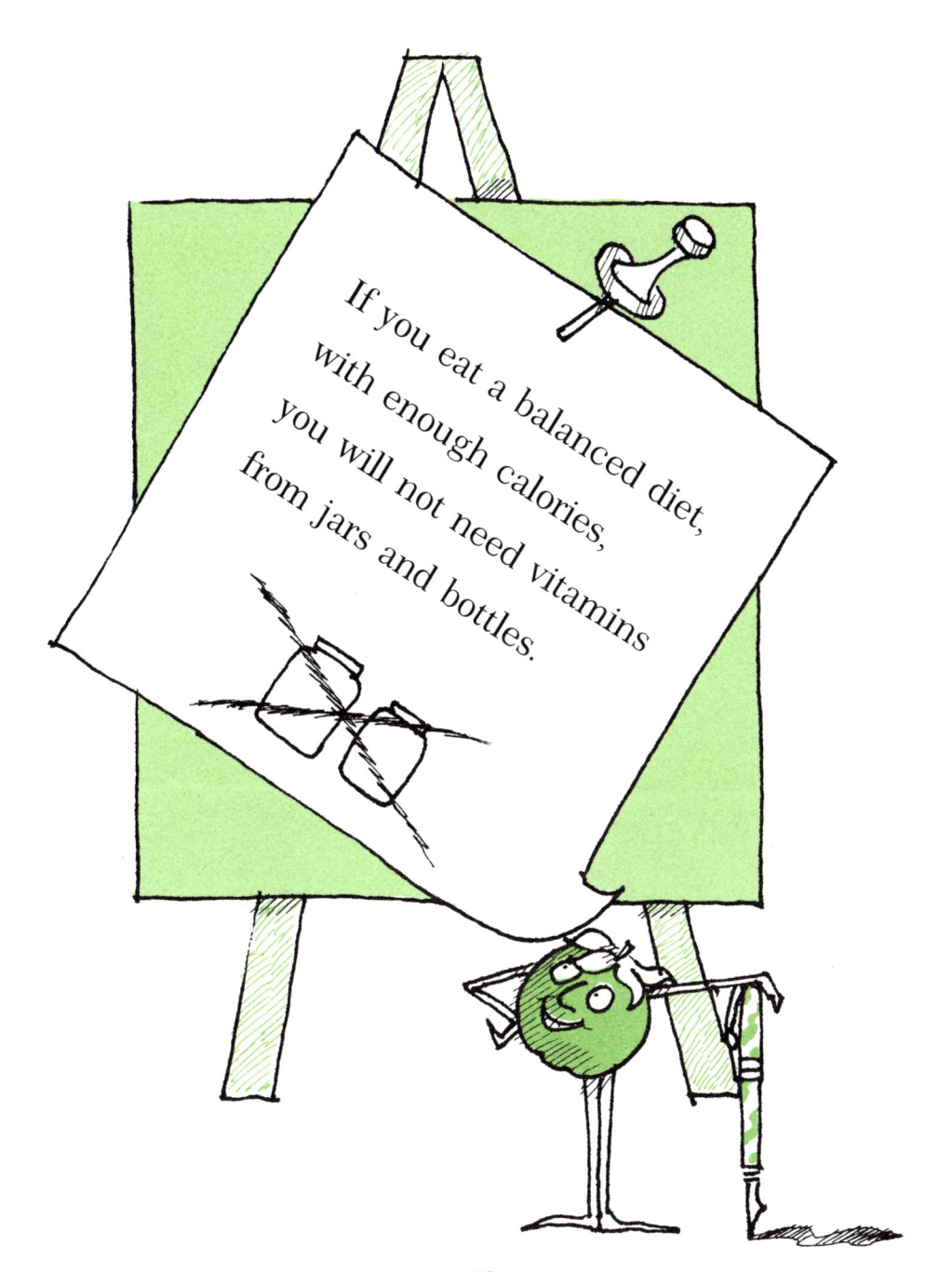

If you eat a balanced diet, with enough calories, you will not need vitamins from jars and bottles.

Who Needs Extra Vitamins?

There are some people who need more vitamins than others. Young children need more vitamins because their bones, teeth, and body tissue are growing fast.

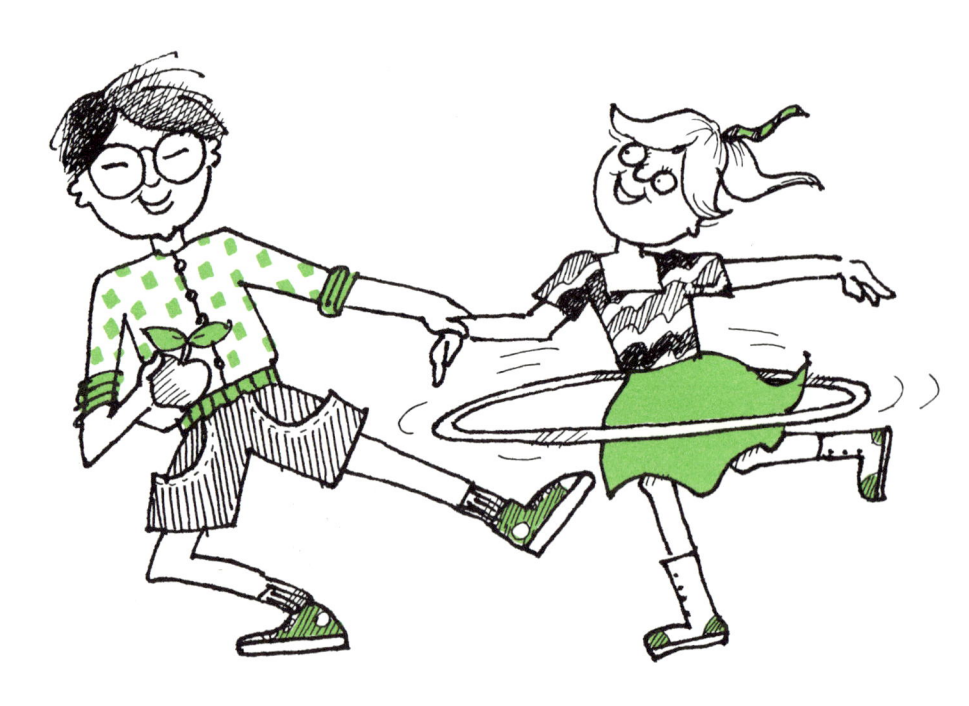

Pregnant women
need more vitamins
because they are eating for
themselves *and* the baby who
is growing inside.

Newborn babies
who are not being
nursed need more vitamins.
They may not be getting all
they need from what they are fed.

People who want to lose weight
may not be eating a balanced diet.
They need extra vitamins.
Alcohol and tobacco make the
body less able to absorb
certain vitamins.
So people who smoke
or drink a lot
need extra vitamins.

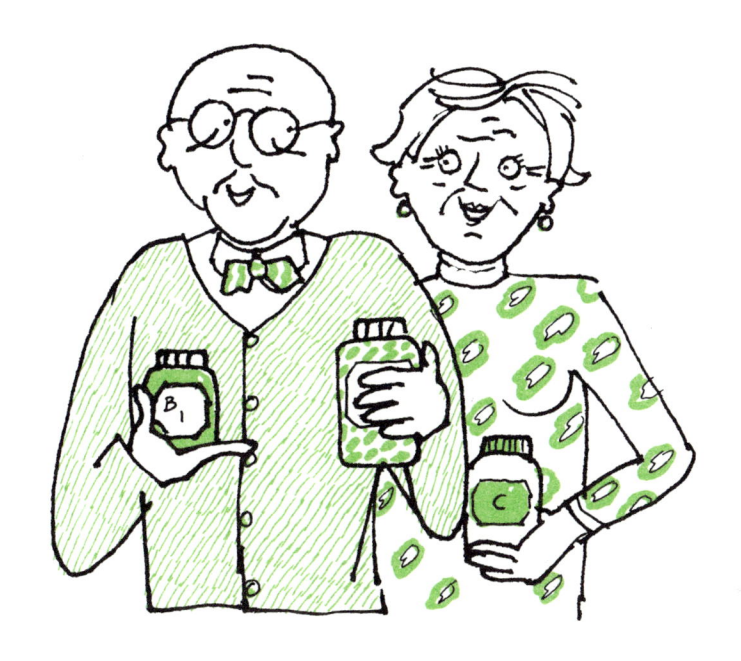

Older people sometimes need extra Vitamin B$_1$ and Vitamin C because their bodies don't absorb enough of these vitamins.
In other words, not everyone needs exactly the same amount of each vitamin.

Conclusion

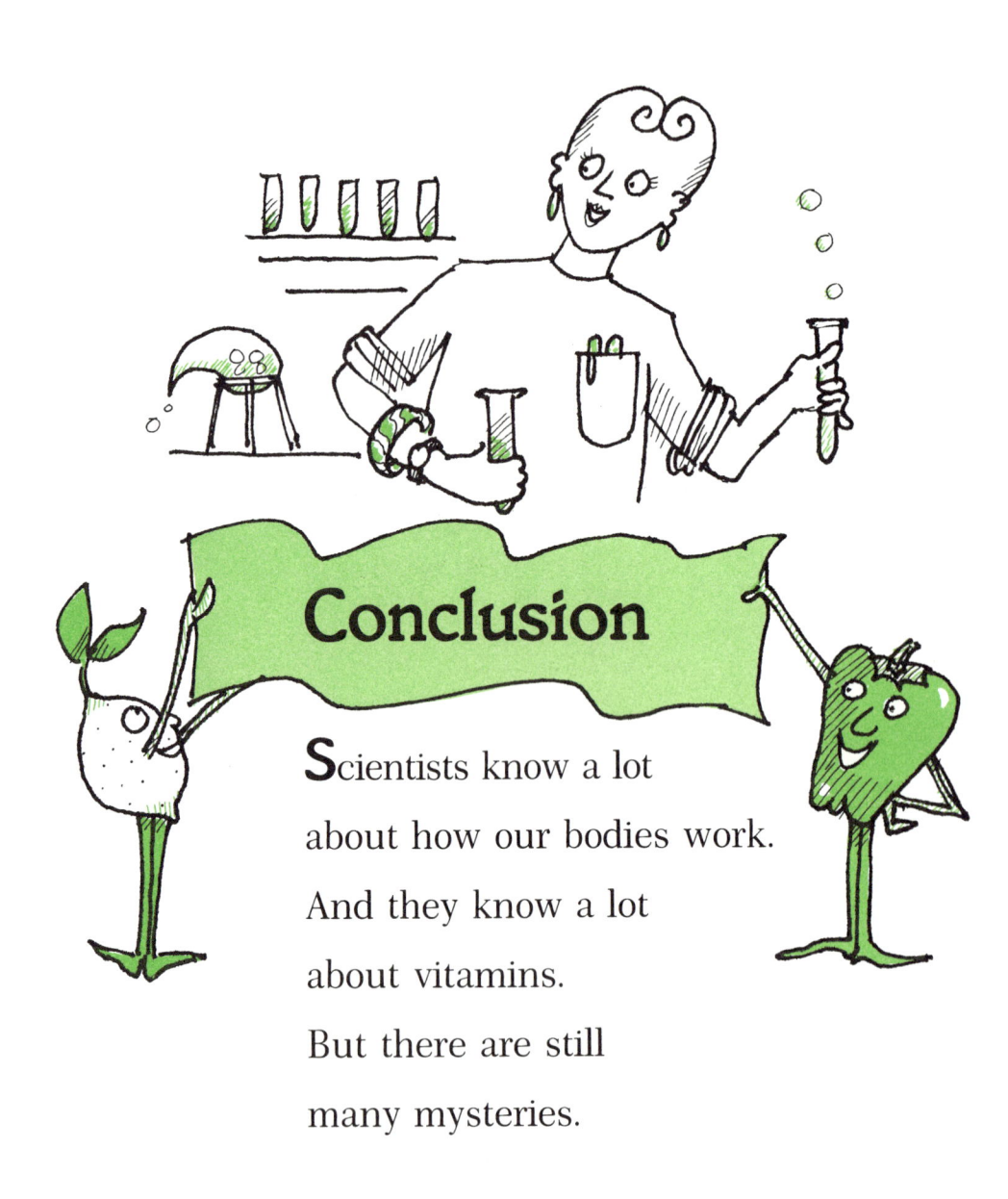

Scientists know a lot about how our bodies work. And they know a lot about vitamins. But there are still many mysteries.

The vitamin team
may not be complete.
If there are undiscovered vitamins,
what do they do?
Some questions may be answered
when we find out more about
how vitamins work together.
Others may be answered
when we know how vitamins
team up with minerals
and other nutrients.
The search goes on!

Now you know why you need
all the vitamins.

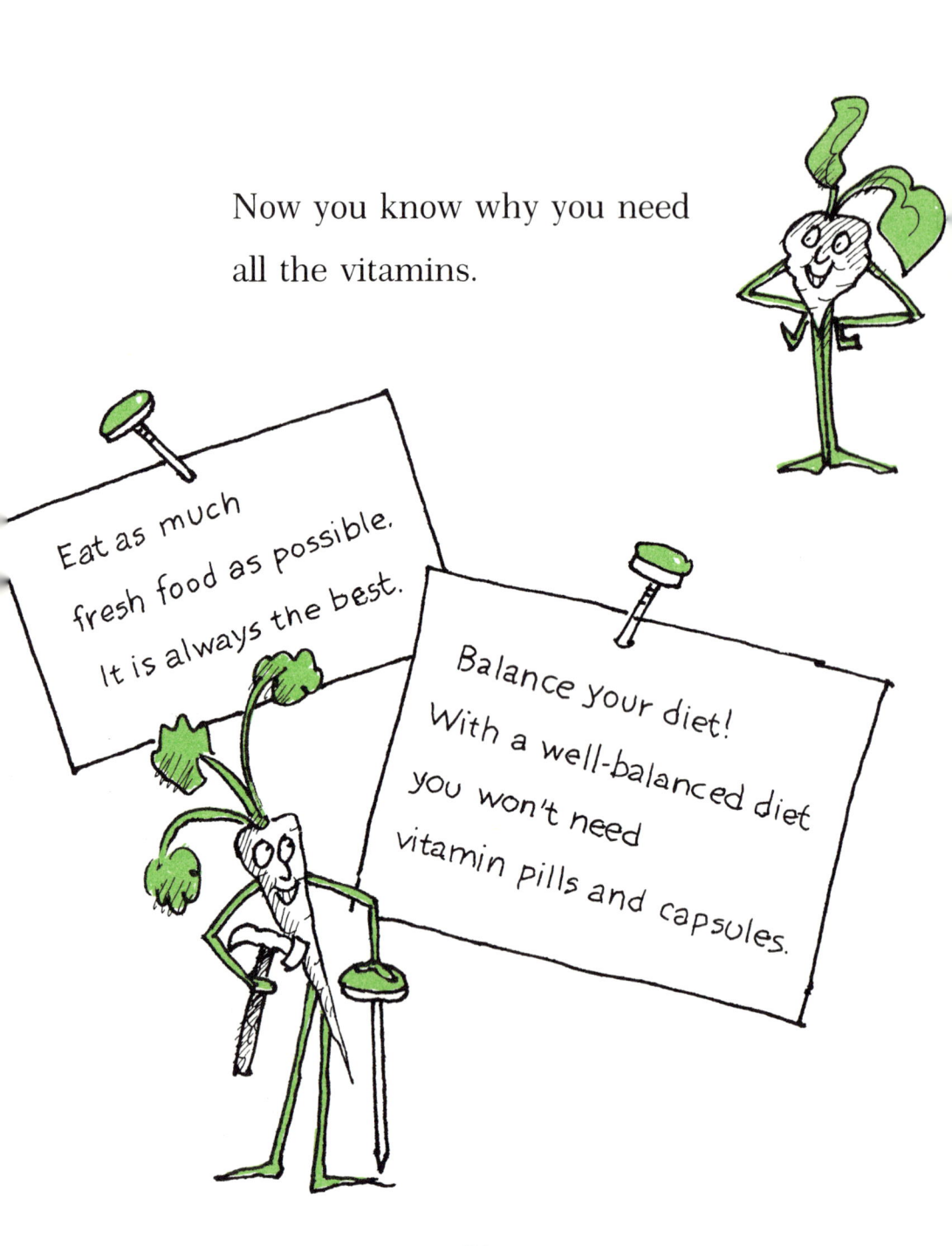

Eat as much fresh food as possible. It is always the best.

Balance your diet! With a well-balanced diet you won't need vitamin pills and capsules.

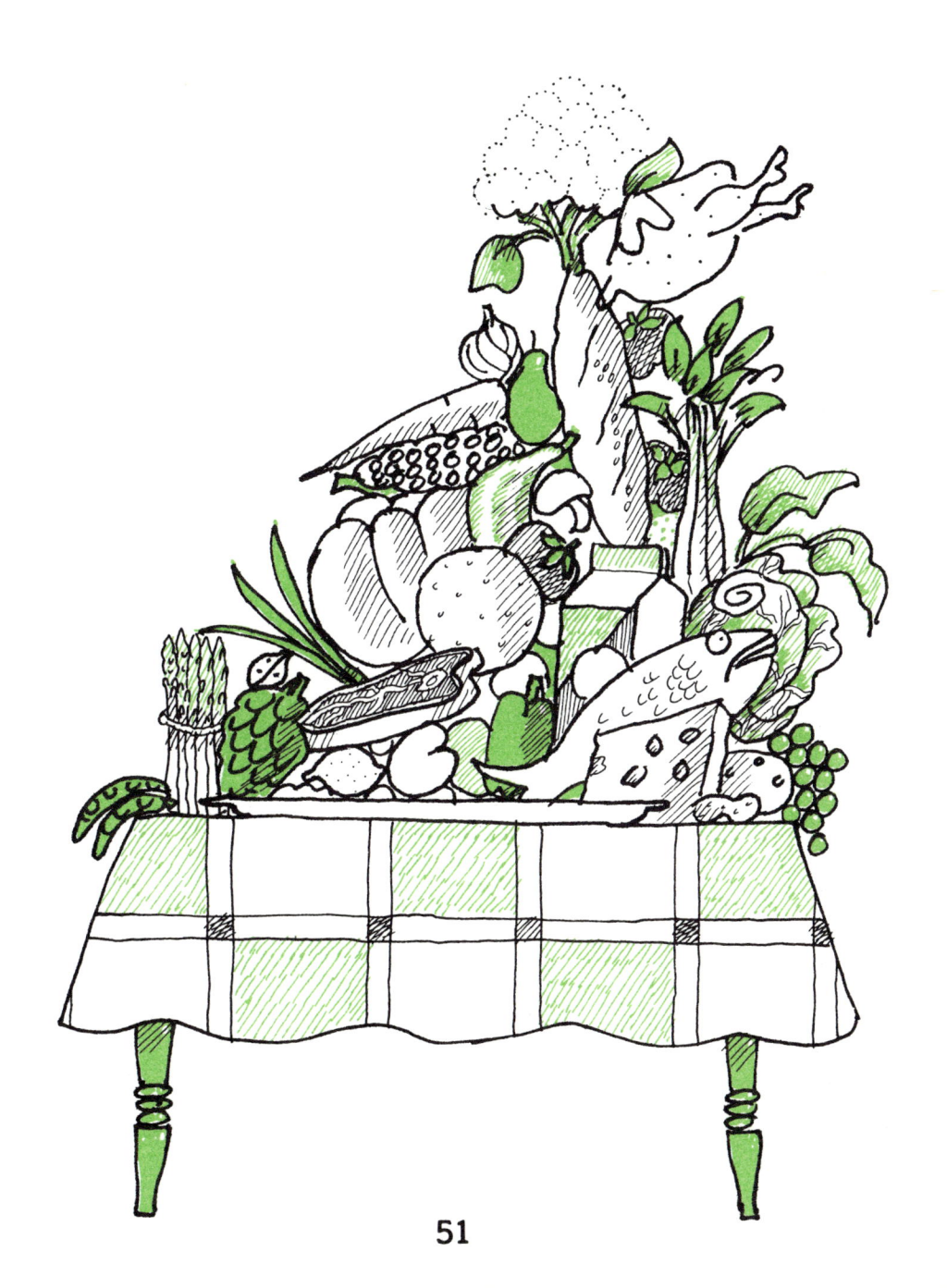

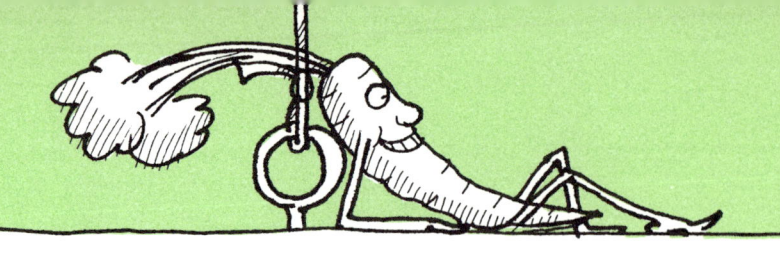

Vitamin Chart

VITAMIN	FOUND IN
A	carrots, sweet potatoes, egg yolks, yellow vegetables
B_1 THIAMINE	ham, lima beans, cereals, liver, oysters
B_2 RIBOFLAVIN	milk, meat, fish, eggs, cheese, vegetables
B_3 NIACIN	meat, fish, egg yolks, grains, green vegetables
B_6 PYRIDOXINE	peanut butter, chicken, fish, potatoes, bananas, green vegetables
B_{12} COBALOMINE	liver, fish, eggs, milk

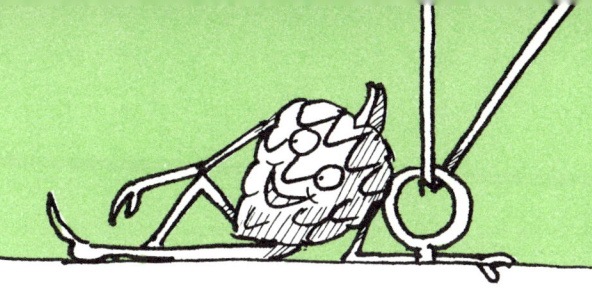

BIOTIN	egg yolks, green vegetables, milk
PANTOTHENIC ACID	almost all plant and animal foods
FOLIC ACID	liver, leafy vegetables, wheat germ, egg yolks, apricots
C	citrus fruits, tomatoes, strawberries, melons, potatoes, green vegetables
D	milk, fish oils, tuna fish, sardines, salmon
E	milk, vegetable oils, potatoes, liver, cabbage, cereals
K	green vegetables, potatoes, liver, cereals, egg yolks

Vitamin Test

TRUE OR FALSE

1.

Dogs and cats need vitamins.

TRUE. All animals need vitamins to grow and stay healthy.

2.

If you take vitamin pills, it doesn't matter what you eat.

FALSE. You must have all the nutrients—fats, proteins, carbohydrates, minerals, and water. You also must have fiber.

3.

You must eat spinach to get enough Vitamin K.

FALSE. There is plenty of Vitamin K in yogurt, egg yolks, and other green vegetables as well.

4.

Colorful vitamin pills are the best.

FALSE. The color is added.
The vitamins in the pills are
what count.

5.

Eggs, milk, liver, whole wheat bread,
and spinach together have
all the vitamins you need.

TRUE. These foods together
have them all.
But you might get bored
if you ate nothing else.

6.

Large doses of Vitamin C
will keep colds away.

FALSE. They may not hurt.
But don't count on Vitamin C
to cure a cold.

JUDITH S. SEIXAS was graduated from Carleton College and has an M.A. from Columbia's Teachers College. She has long been involved in health issues, specializing in the treatment of alcoholics and their families. Her wide experience encompasses both the educational and the therapeutic. She is the co-author of *Children of Alcoholism: A Survivor's Manual* and for children the author of: *Junk Food—What It Is, What It Does, Alcohol—What It Is, What It Does, Tobacco—What It Is, What It Does,* and *Living with a Parent Who Drinks too Much.*

TOM HUFFMAN attended the School of Visual Arts in New York City and holds a B.A. from the University of Kentucky. Mr. Huffman is a free-lance artist whose works have appeared in galleries, advertisements, and national magazines. He has illustrated many children's books including five Greenwillow Read-alone Books.

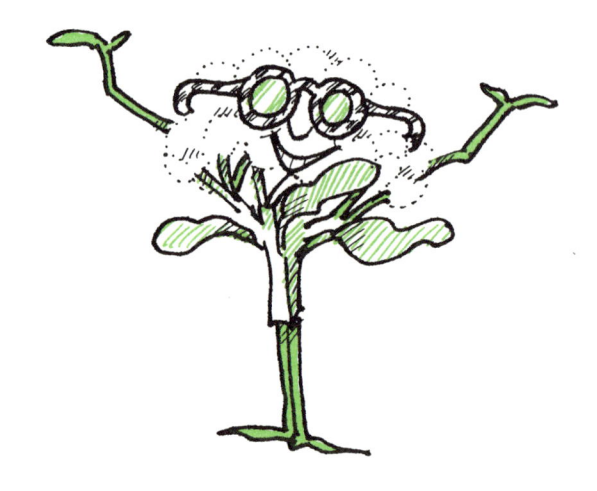